HIGH-PROTEIN

SHAKES

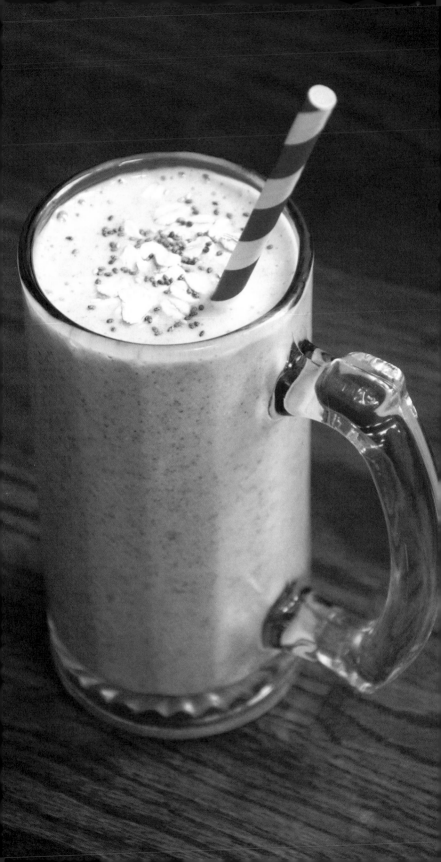

PAMELA BRAUN

HIGH-PROTEIN

SHAKES

STRENGTH-BUILDING RECIPES
FOR EVERYDAY HEALTH

THE COUNTRYMAN PRESS

A division of W. W. Norton & Company

Independent Publishers Since 1923

For information about permission to reproduce selections
from this book, write to Permissions, The Countryman Press,
500 Fifth Avenue, New York, NY 10110

For information about special discounts for bulk purchases, please
contact W. W. Norton Special Sales at specialsales@wwnorton.com
or 800-233-4830

Book design by Chin-Yee Lai
Manufacturing by Versa Press
Production manager: Devon Zahn

The Countryman Press
www.countrymanpress.com

A division of W. W. Norton & Company, Inc.
500 Fifth Avenue, New York, N.Y. 10110
www.wwnorton.com

978-1-682-68025-4 (pbk.)

10   9   8   7   6   5   4   3   2   1

CONTENTS

Protein isn't just for weight lifters and gym rats. Protein helps to keep you feeling full longer and it supports building bones and muscles.

Are you looking for a delicious way to get more protein in your diet or are you bored with your current go-to shakes? This book will assist you in finding more delicious ways to get that protein you're looking for or shake up your current shake routine.

EQUIPMENT

I use a high-speed blender when I make these shakes. I find that there's less blending time and the ingredients break down and blend better—but you can use a regular blender or one of those smaller, high-speed bullet–type blenders to make these shakes. The only thing about the smaller blenders to keep in mind is that not all of the ingredients may fit in the container. You may need to get a bigger container to hold all of the ingredients.

INGREDIENTS

The ingredients I use in these shakes are easy to find at your local grocery or health food store. I want these high-protein shakes to be as simple to make as possible.

FRUITS

The best fruit you can use is fresh fruit, either in season or that you cut up and froze yourself. Of course that's not always possible to do. In that case, try different brands of frozen fruit until you find one that has great flavor (they're not all the same) and use that product.

Several of these recipes call for ripe bananas. Whenever possible, use bananas with brown spots on them. The brown spots mean that the banana is sweeter than that of bright yellow skinned bananas. Using the bright yellow skinned bananas in shakes can lead to a bland or less sweet-tasting shake. Since many of these recipes don't call for added sweeteners, this can mean the shake will taste very different from what was intended.

PROTEIN POWDER

Not many of the shakes call for protein powder, but a few do. Beyond the various flavors available in protein powders, there are many different types of protein powders. Which one is right for you? Maybe there's more than one kind.

There are basically two categories of protein powders: animal-derived protein powders (egg and whey) and vegetable protein powders (rice, pea, hemp, and soy).

Animal-based protein powders are said to be absorbed and utilized by the body easier than vegetable-based protein powders, but both are good. It's really up to you and your dietary requirements which one you choose to use.

An important thing to consider with protein powders is sweetened or unsweetened. The recipes in this book that call for protein powders let you know if it should be unsweetened. If the recipe simply calls for protein powder (vanilla or chocolate are the flavors used in this book), then how it is sweetened is up to you. Protein powders are sweetened with artificial or natural sweeteners as well as artificial or natural flavorings. There are enough protein powders on the market that you should be able to find your preference.

The other consideration when choosing a protein powder is the amount of protein in each serving. This can vary widely.

Protein shakes can be a smart food choice if you're trying to lose weight, build muscle, or are just looking for a snack or meal replacement. This is especially applicable if you make the shake yourself and you know exactly what's gone into it.

LIQUID INGREDIENTS

For these shakes I use coconut milk (the full-fat milk that comes in a can), coconut water, 2% milk, and cashew milk. Once you open the can of coconut milk, the leftover can be stored in a covered container in the refrigerator. When you are ready to use the leftover milk, make sure that you stir it well as the fat tends to separate from the liquid.

I use the 2% milk for extra protein and cashew milk because I like the thicker consistency that it has. However, you could use any nut/soy milk you like in place of the cashew milk. You could even use 2% milk in place of the nut/soy milk.

BLENDING TIME

The time it takes to fully blend your shake depends on what type of blender you are using. But when blending the shake ingredients, you want to blend until everything is fully incorporated into the shake. Even with the high-speed blender, I keep it running for at least a minute and a half.

NUTRITIONAL INFORMATION

The nutritional information listed with each shake is an approximation. Values will change based on the protein powder that you use and/or any ingredient substitutions that you may make (e.g. using whole milk instead of 2% milk). They can also differ with the measurement of frozen fruit, which is definitely not an exact science.

Each of these recipes makes one shake.

Enjoy the fresh, delicious, and healthy shake you just made!

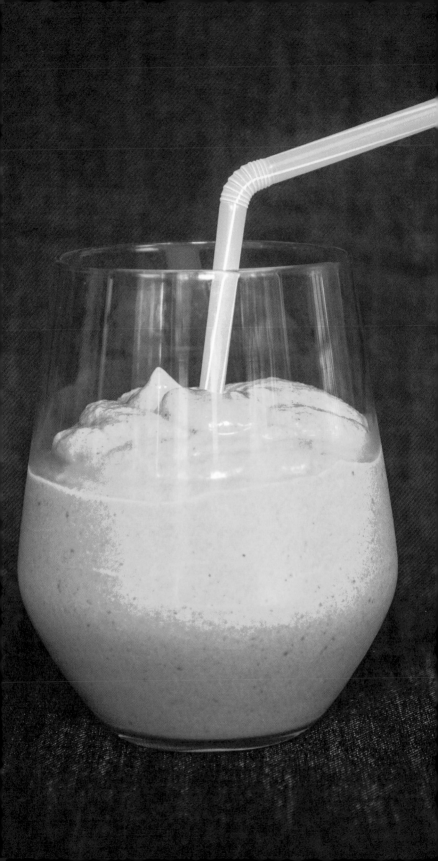

PUMPKIN SPICE SHAKE

½ cup pumpkin puree, frozen
and broken into pieces
¼ cup cannellini beans, drained
and rinsed
5.3 ounces vanilla Greek yogurt
½ teaspoon ground allspice

½ teaspoon ground cinnamon
½ teaspoon ground ginger
1 tablespoon hemp hearts
1 pitted date, chopped
¼ cup ice water

1. To freeze the pumpkin you need to measure it out, then
   put it into a zip-top bag. Close the bag, then spread the
   pumpkin into a thin layer. Put the bag in the freezer
   overnight.
2. When ready to make the shake, break up the pumpkin
   by lightly hitting the pumpkin with a rolling pin.
3. Add all ingredients to a blender and blend until smooth.
4. Pour into glass.
5. Serve.

Protein 23 grams | Carbs 48 grams | Calories 184

Pumpkin spice flavored everything is huge
in the fall, but why does it have to be for fall
only? This cool and creamy shake brings
you all of your favorite autumn flavors any
time of the year. You can dress this up with
a sprinkling of hemp seeds and cinnamon
on top if you're feeling fancy.

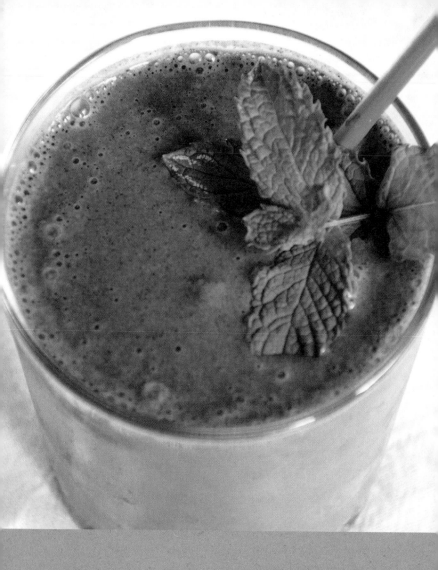

The green monster might sound scary, but it's definitely not. The vanilla sweet-ness from the yogurt, the banana, and the creamy almond butter are what you taste in this smooth shake. Not only does the spirulina add to the gorgeous green hue of this drink, but it also gives you an omega-3 boost, a hit of chlorophyll, and lots of other healthy nutrients.

GREEN MONSTER SHAKE

GREEN MONSTER
SHAKE

5.3 ounces vanilla Greek yogurt

1 medium banana, cut into chunks and frozen

1 tablespoon organic spirulina powder

1 tablespoon hemp powder

1 tablespoon creamy almond butter

¾ cup unsweetened cashew milk

1. Add all ingredients to a blender and blend until smooth.
2. Pour into glass.
3. Serve.

Protein 28 grams | Carbs 49 grams | Calories 293

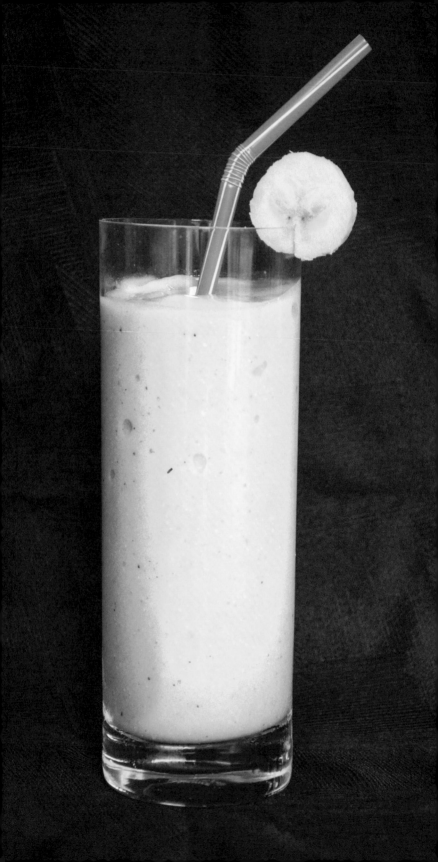

TROPICAL SHAKE

½ cup cannellini beans, drained
  and rinsed
1 tablespoon hemp hearts
½ cup frozen pineapple chunks
⅔ cup frozen mango

½ medium banana, cut into
  chunks and frozen
1 cup coconut water
2 tablespoons maca powder

1. Add all ingredients to a blender and blend until smooth.
2. Pour into glass.
3. Serve.

Protein 14 grams | Carbs 64 grams | Calories 307

Let's take a trip to the tropics! This tropical shake will have you forgetting all about how much protein you're getting and whisk you away to a faraway island. The not-too-tart, not-too-sweet flavors of this shake are melded perfectly by the cannellini beans and banana.

BANANA WHIP SHAKE

10 raw almonds
½ cup silken tofu
1 medium banana, cut into
    chunks and frozen
2 tablespoons old-fashioned
    rolled oats

1 tablespoon flax seed
2 pitted dates, chopped
¼ teaspoon cinnamon
¾ cup coconut water

1. Add all ingredients to a blender and blend until smooth.
2. Pour into glass.
3. Serve.

Protein 17 grams | Carbs 85 grams | Calories 505

This refreshing shake has the smooth flavor of banana but is so light and airy you'll be surprised by how filling it is. There's a good punch of protein hiding in this shake too, so it will stay with you for a long time and won't give you those dreaded ups and downs.

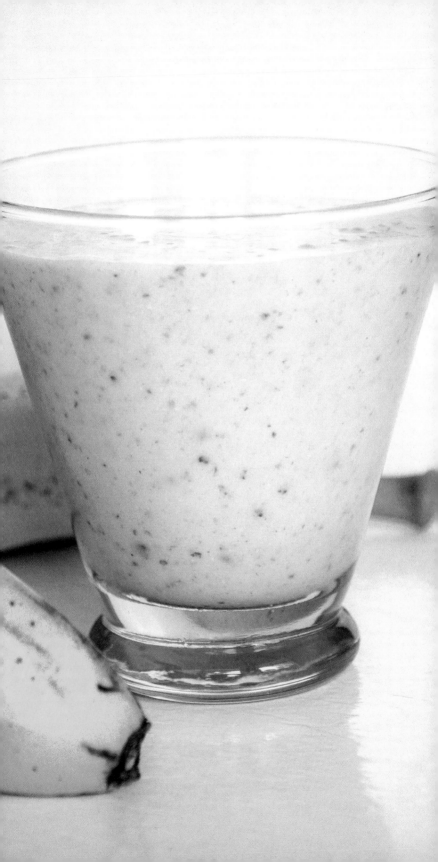

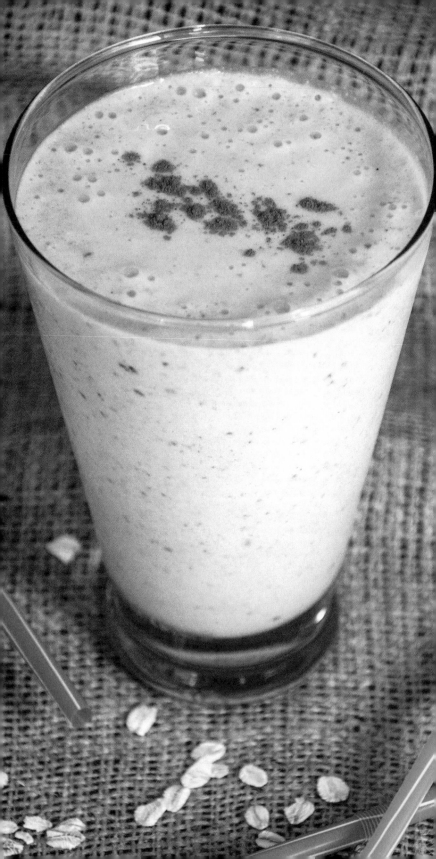

OATMEAL COOKIE SHAKE

10 raw almonds
½ cup silken tofu
1 medium banana, cut into
    chunks and frozen
2 tablespoons old-fashioned
    rolled oats

1 tablespoon flax seed
1 pitted date, chopped
¼ teaspoon cinnamon
¾ cup unsweetened cashew
    milk

1. Add all ingredients to a blender and blend until smooth.
2. Pour into glass.
3. Serve.

Protein 17 grams | Carbs 61 grams | Calories 424

It's like you put a bunch of oatmeal cookies in a blender and let it go. The Oatmeal Cookie Shake has all the flavors of an oatmeal cookie but in a slightly more refreshing—and definitely better for you—form. A rich and creamy shake will keep you full for quite a while and satisfy your sweet craving at the same time.

STRAWBERRY ORANGE SHAKE

5.3 ounces plain Greek yogurt
2 tablespoons chia seeds
1 tablespoon hemp hearts
1 cup frozen strawberries

1 navel orange, peeled and
de-seeded
½ cup coconut water

1. Add all ingredients to a blender and blend until smooth.
2. Pour into glass.
3. Serve.

Protein 28 grams | Carbs 53 grams | Calories 303

Looking for a way to wake up in the morning without your usual coffee? This shake will definitely do it. It's got the bright flavors of strawberry, orange, and Greek yogurt to perk up your taste buds and make you take notice. This shake comes together really quickly too, so you won't be late for work.

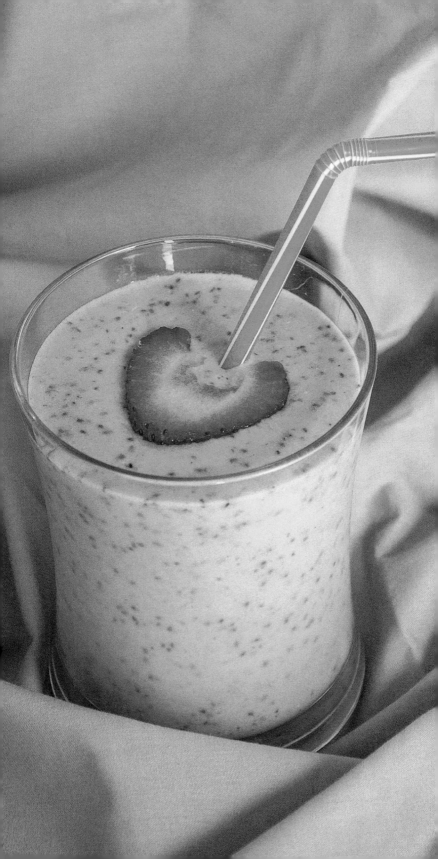

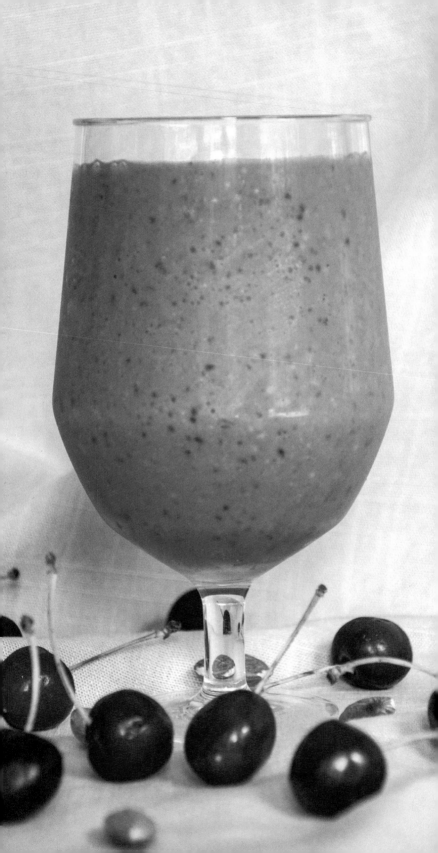

CHERRY ALMOND SHAKE

1 cup cherries, pitted and frozen
5.3 ounces plain Greek yogurt
½ cup silken tofu
⅛ teaspoon almond extract
10 raw almonds

1 tablespoon hemp hearts
2 tablespoons old-fashioned
    rolled oats
¾ cup unsweetened cashew
    milk

1. Add all ingredients to a blender and blend until smooth.
2. Pour into glass.
3. Serve.

Protein 28 grams | Carbs 38 grams | Calories 248

When cherry met almond, it was love at first sight. Cherries have a subtle flavor that comes out a bit more when paired with almonds. This shake will give you lots of protein while you're sipping on its sweetness.

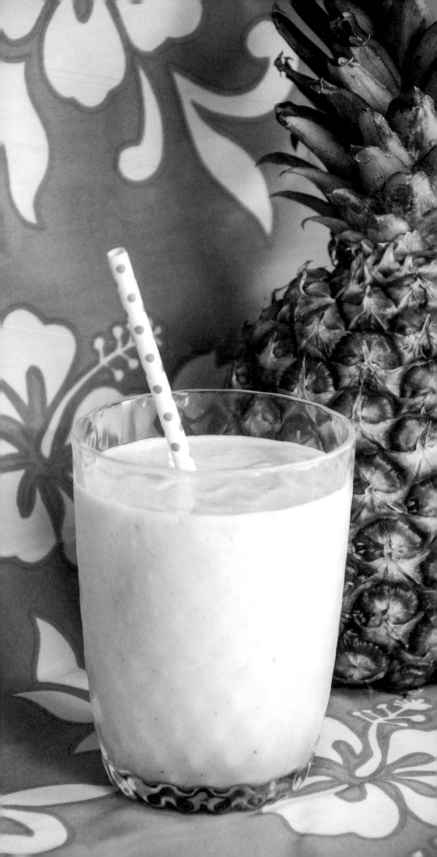

PIÑA COLADA SHAKE

¼ cup raw cashews, soaked in water overnight
½ cup low-fat 2% cottage cheese
1 tablespoon hemp hearts

½ generous cup frozen pineapple chunks
¼ cup canned coconut milk
½ cup coconut water

---

1. Drain cashews.
2. Add all ingredients to a blender and blend until smooth.
3. Pour into glass.
4. Serve.

Protein 27 grams | Carbs 34 grams | Calories 514

The tropics are calling with this Piña Colada Shake. The flavors of coconut and pineapple come through and there's a good shot of protein from the cottage cheese and cashews too. So why not take a few minutes to daydream about wiggling your toes in the sand while you enjoy this healthy treat?

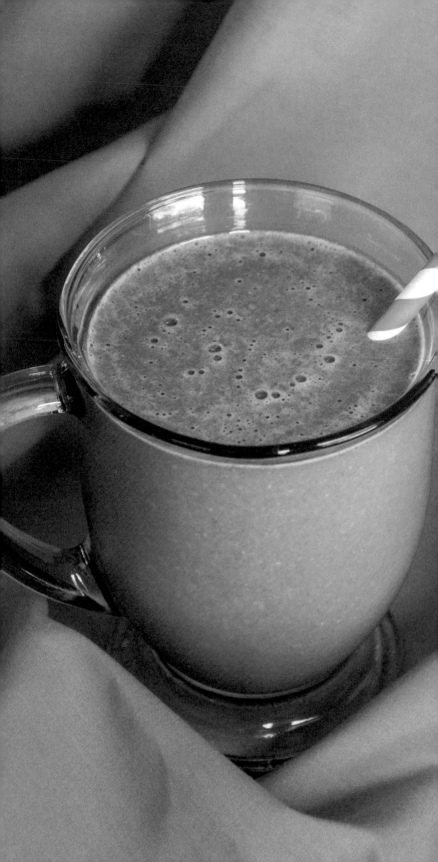

MEXICAN CHOCOLATE SHAKE

5.3 ounces plain Greek yogurt
10 raw almonds
¼ cup cooked quinoa, chilled
1½ tablespoons unsweetened
   cocoa powder
½ teaspoon cinnamon

1 medium banana, cut into
   chunks and frozen
¾ cup unsweetened cashew
   milk
1 tablespoon maple syrup
   (optional)

1. Add all ingredients to a blender and blend until smooth.
2. Pour into glass.
3. Serve.

Protein 25 grams | Carbs 64 grams | Calories 334

Mexican hot chocolate is delicious with its rich chocolate flavor and hint of spice. This shake version makes things cold and refreshing on a hot day. For a bit of sweetness, add some maple syrup, or go bold and add a dash of heat with some cayenne.

PEANUT BUTTER OATMEAL SHAKE

1 medium banana, cut into
  chunks and frozen
¼ cup powdered peanut butter
2 tablespoons old-fashioned
  rolled oats

1 tablespoon chia seeds
2 tablespoons egg white
  powder
¾ cup unsweetened cashew
  milk

1. Add all ingredients to a blender and blend until smooth.
2. Pour into glass.
3. Serve.

Protein 32 grams | Carbs 62 grams | Calories 422

This thick and creamy Peanut Butter Oatmeal Shake is loaded with peanutty goodness. It gets its creaminess from the banana and more flavor and protein from the oats. This shake comes together really quickly so you can whip up this shake and be on your way in no time.

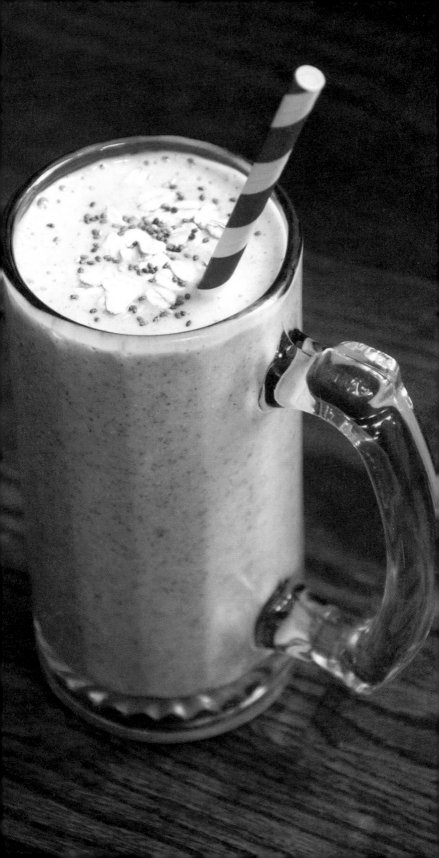

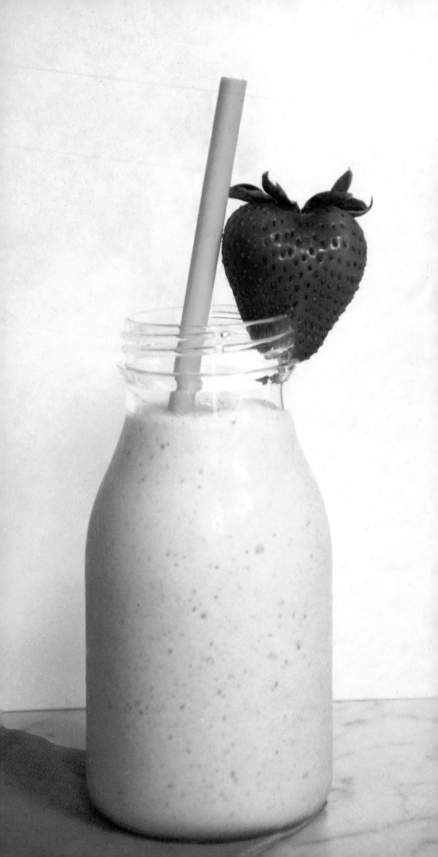

STRAWBERRY CHEESECAKE SHAKE

1 cup frozen strawberries
½ cup low-fat 2% cottage
  cheese

1 tablespoon egg white powder
1 teaspoon vanilla extract
½ cup 2% milk

---

1. Add all ingredients to a blender and blend until smooth.
2. Pour into glass.
3. Serve.

Protein 25 grams | Carbs 20 grams | Calories 216

Who doesn't love a big piece of strawberry cheesecake? But then you have all the fat and calories to deal with afterward. This cool and creamy Strawberry Cheesecake Shake gives you the flavor of cheesecake with lots of good-for-you ingredients minus the guilt.

RASPBERRY ALMOND SHAKE

5.3 ounces plain Greek yogurt
½ cup frozen raspberries
1 tablespoon maple syrup
1 tablespoon chia seeds

1 tablespoon hemp hearts
⅛ teaspoon almond extract
½ cup unsweetened cashew
  milk

1. Add all ingredients to a blender and blend until smooth.
2. Pour into glass.
3. Serve.

Protein 27 grams | Carbs 37 grams | Calories 273

Start your day with the sweet, tart flavor of raspberries. This Raspberry Almond Shake provides protein, fiber, and good-for-you fats to keep you satisfied all morning long. The Greek yogurt brings out the tart side of the raspberries and the maple syrup helps to bring out their sweeter side. The combination of the two will make your taste buds sing.

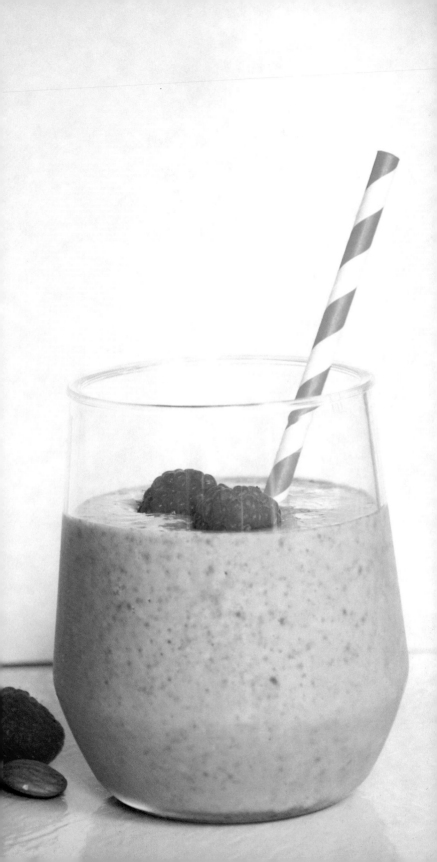

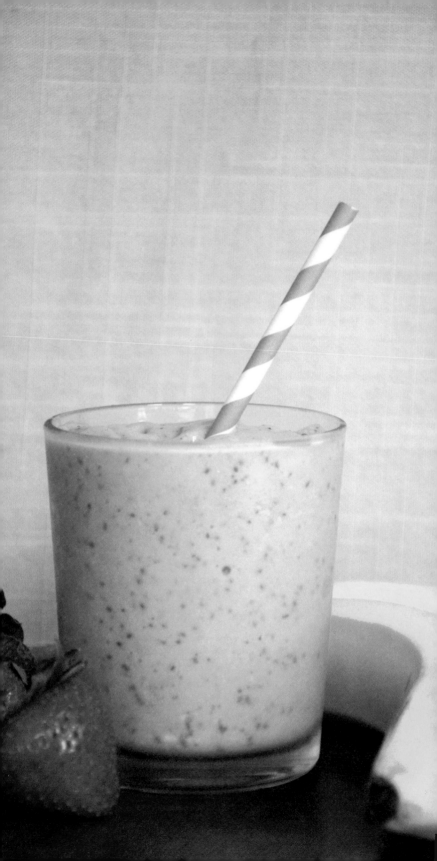

STRAWBERRY BANANA SHAKE

1 cup frozen strawberries
1 medium banana, cut into
   chunks and frozen
½ cup silken tofu

1 tablespoon chia seeds
1 tablespoon hemp hearts
1 cup unsweetened cashew
   milk

1. Add all ingredients to a blender and blend until smooth.
2. Pour into glass.
3. Serve.

Protein 19 grams | Carbs 49 grams | Calories 351

Strawberries and bananas have gone together forever. Zingy strawberries paired with mellow bananas make a flavor combination that's hard to beat. Throw in all those great protein-filled ingredients and you've got yourself a shake that's healthy and delicious.

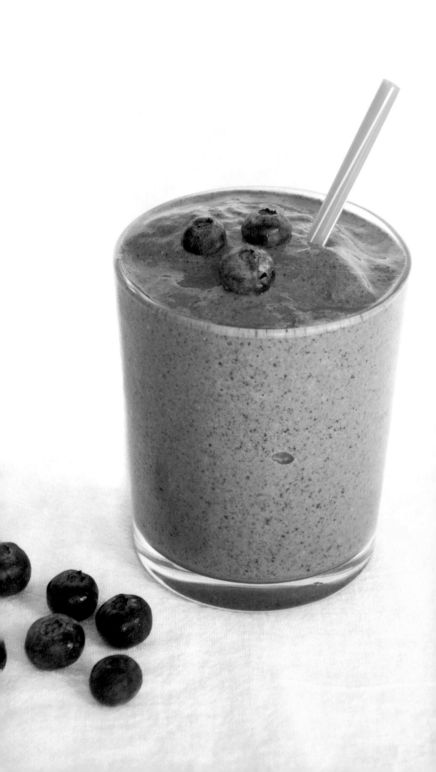

BLUEBERRY MANGO SHAKE

½ cup frozen blueberries
½ cup frozen mangoes
½ cup low-fat 2% cottage
   cheese

1 tablespoon chia seeds
1 tablespoon hemp seeds
½ cup unsweetened cashew
   milk

1. Add all ingredients to a blender and blend until smooth.
2. Pour into glass.
3. Serve.

Protein 23 grams | Carbs 33 grams | Calories 279

Blueberries and mangoes might come from very different places, but they sure do play nicely together. These two fruits come together in a shake that's not only loaded with protein, it's also loaded with lots of fruit flavor and antioxidants.

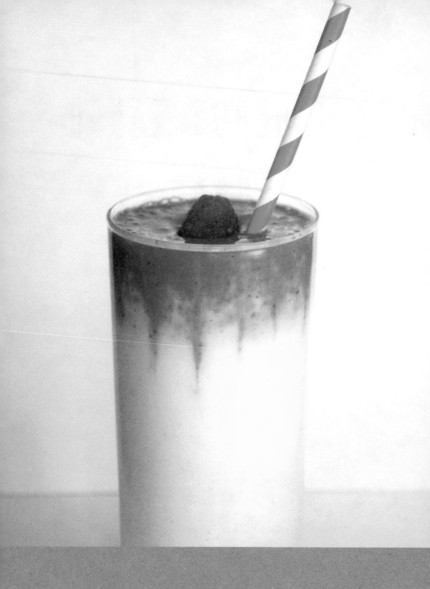

Sometimes you just can't make up your mind. Do you want raspberry in your shake or pineapple? This layered shake gives you the best of both worlds. This shake has lots of protein in it since it's got a good bit in each of the layers. As an added bonus, it's also really pretty.

RASPBERRY PINEAPPLE SHAKE

RASPBERRY PINEAPPLE SHAKE

Pineapple Layer
¾ cup frozen pineapple chunks
½ cup cannellini beans, drained
  and rinsed
¼ cup silken tofu
1 tablespoon egg white powder
½ cup unsweetened cashew milk

Raspberry Layer
¾ cup frozen raspberries
¼ cup cannellini beans, drained
  and rinsed
¼ cup silken tofu
½ cup unsweetened cashew
  milk

1. Add the ingredients for the pineapple layer to a blender and blend until smooth. Pour into a glass.
2. Clean out the blender then add the ingredients for the raspberry layer to the blender and blend until smooth. Pour on top of the pineapple mixture in the glass.
3. To make the raspberry stream through the pineapple layer, use a straw to poke the raspberry down into the pineapple layer.
4. Serve.

Protein 15 grams | Carbs 39 grams | Calories 254

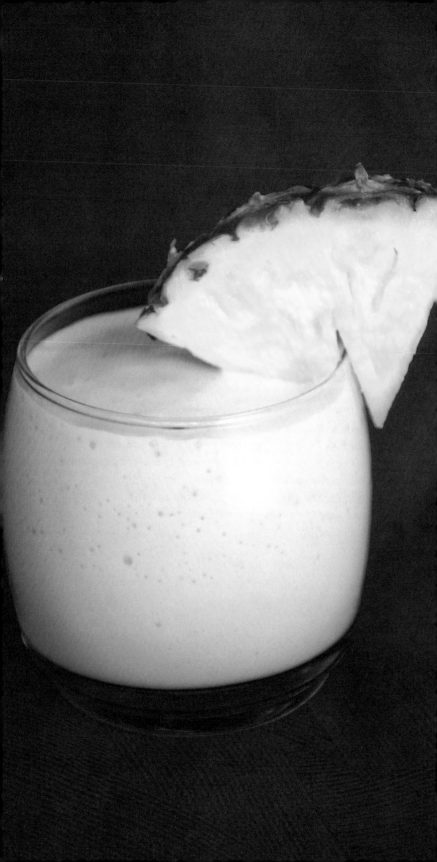

PINEAPPLE WHIP SHAKE

1½ cups frozen pineapple
chunks
½ cup low-fat 2% cottage
cheese

½ cup silken tofu
½ cup unsweetened cashew
milk

1. Add all ingredients to a blender and blend until smooth.
2. Pour into glass.
3. Serve.

Protein 24 grams | Carbs 34 grams | Calories 275

If you like pineapple Dole whips, you're really going to like this high-protein version. It's got that same lip-smacking pineapple flavor, but with a good amount of protein to keep you going longer. Since it only has four ingredients, it's a snap to whip together too.

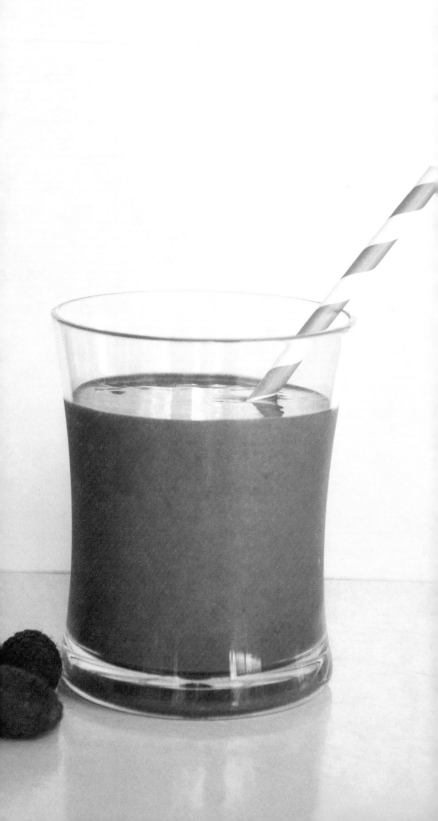

CHOCOLATE RASPBERRY SHAKE

5.3 ounces plain Greek yogurt
¾ cup frozen raspberries
1 tablespoon chia seeds
1 tablespoon unsweetened
  cocoa powder

1 tablespoon maple syrup
½ cup unsweetened cashew
  milk

1. Add all ingredients to a blender and blend until smooth.
2. Pour into glass.
3. Serve.

Protein 21 grams | Carbs 39 grams | Calories 192

Need a chocolate fix, but don't want that crash you get from eating a chocolate bar? This Chocolate Raspberry Shake is exactly what you need. With 20-plus grams of protein, this shake will help get you through that afternoon lull.

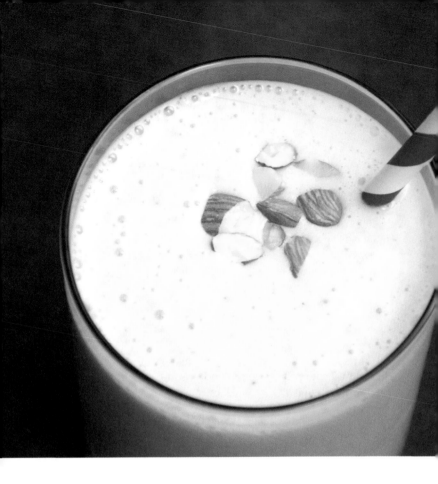

VANILLA ALMOND
SHAKE

5.3 ounces vanilla Greek yogurt
10 raw almonds
1 medium banana, cut into
　chunks and frozen

1 tablespoon maca powder
¼ teaspoon almond extract
½ cup unsweetened cashew
　milk

44

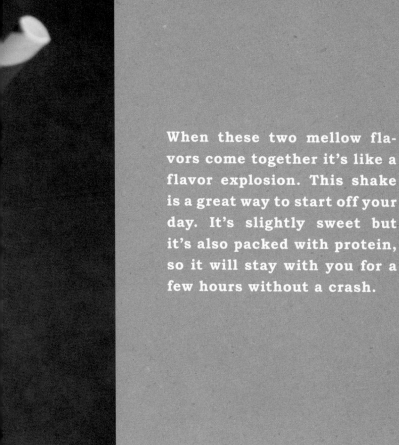

When these two mellow flavors come together it's like a flavor explosion. This shake is a great way to start off your day. It's slightly sweet but it's also packed with protein, so it will stay with you for a few hours without a crash.

1. Add all ingredients to a blender and blend until smooth.
2. Pour into glass.
3. Serve.

Protein 18 grams | Carbs 45 grams | Calories 204

VANILLA ALMOND SHAKE

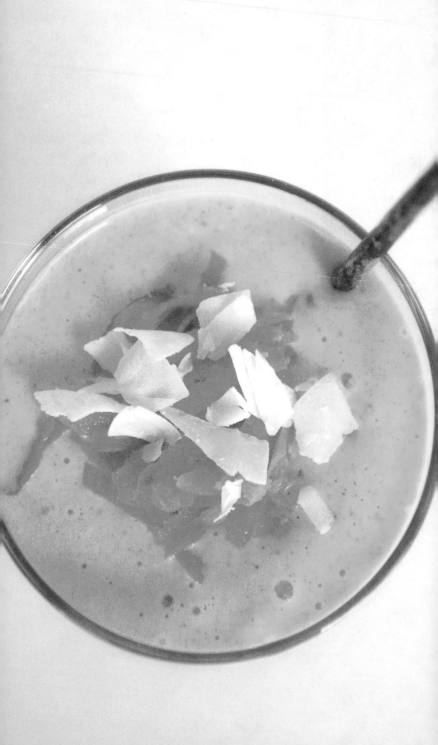

CARROT CAKE SHAKE

1 carrot (3½" long, with a
diameter of approximately 1")
cut into small pieces
¾ cup frozen pineapple chunks
½ cup low-fat 2% cottage
cheese

½ cup silken tofu
2 tablespoons unsweetened
shredded coconut
¼ teaspoon cinnamon
½ cup 2% milk

1. Add all ingredients to a blender and blend until smooth.
2. Pour into glass.
3. Serve.

Protein 28 grams | Carbs 30 grams | Calories 350

Like carrot cake but didn't think you could
get those flavors in a shake without tossing
a piece of cream cheese–laden cake into a
blender, did you? Well, you'll be pleasantly
surprised with the carrot cake flavors that
come through in this healthy shake. The
only thing missing is all the fat and calories
from the cream cheese frosting.

STRAWBERRY PEACH SHAKE

1 cup frozen strawberries
½ cup frozen peaches
½ cup silken tofu
1 tablespoon chia seeds

1 tablespoon hemp hearts
1 tablespoon flax seeds
1 cup unsweetened cashew
milk

1. Add all ingredients to a blender and blend until smooth.
2. Pour into glass.
3. Serve.

Protein 20 grams | Carbs 33 grams | Calories 334

Strawberries and peaches are at their summertime best in this thick and healthy shake. The tanginess of the strawberries blends well with sweet peaches. This shake is perfect for those hot HOT summer days when you need something to cool down and help you get through the day.

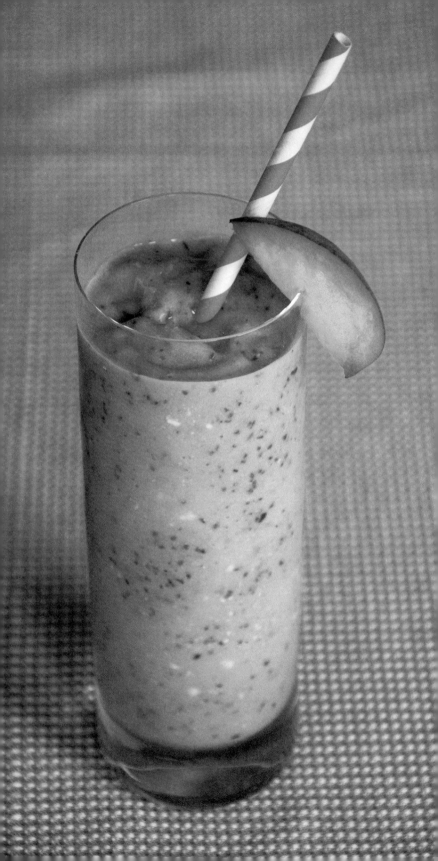

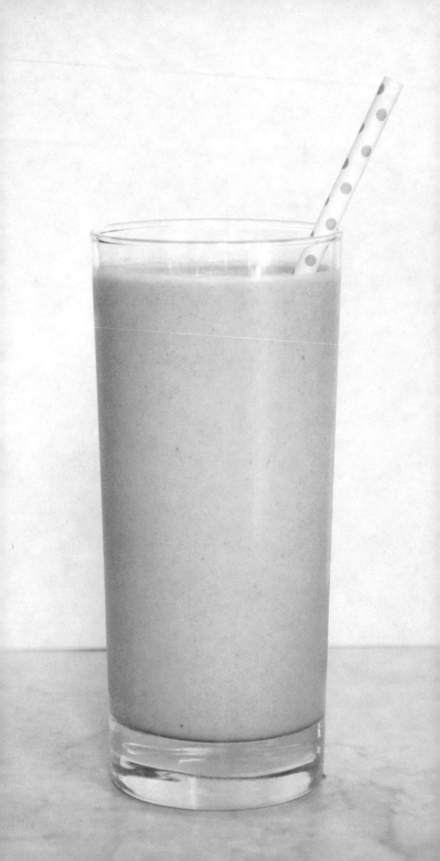

SPINACH BANANA SHAKE

5.3 ounces plain Greek yogurt
1 cup packed baby spinach
1 medium banana, cut into
   chunks and frozen
1 tablespoon hemp powder

1 tablespoon creamy peanut
   butter
¾ cup unsweetened cashew
   milk

1. Add all ingredients to a blender and blend until smooth.
2. Pour into glass.
3. Serve.

Protein 28 grams | Carbs 39 grams | Calories 273

Think all green shakes are the same? Think again! This Spinach Banana Shake has a bit of sweetness from the banana and just a hint of the peanut butter. You won't even taste the spinach in this one. But just because you can't taste it doesn't mean you aren't getting all those good-for-you vitamins and minerals.

SPINACH BANANA SHAKE

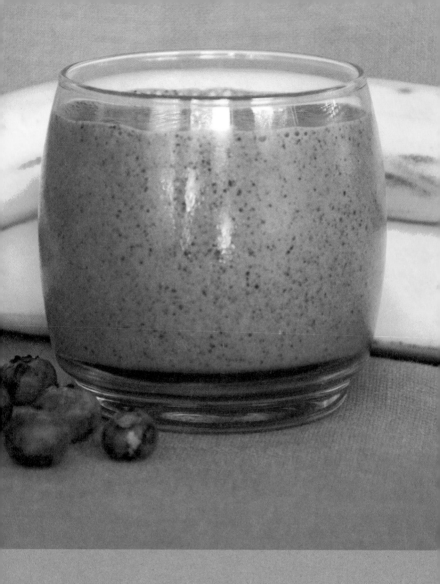

This antioxidant-rich shake is full of great blueberry and banana flavor. Plus it contains more than 10 percent of your daily vitamin C requirement. It has a smooth and mellow flavor from the addition of the cottage cheese and tofu. And with just a few ingredients, it's a great shake to start your day with.

BLUEBERRY BANANA SHAKE

BLUEBERRY BANANA SHAKE

½ cup frozen blueberries
1 medium banana, cut into
  chunks and frozen
½ cup low-fat 2% cottage
  cheese

½ cup silken tofu
½ cup unsweetened cashew
  milk

---

1. Add all ingredients to a blender and blend until smooth.
2. Pour into glass.
3. Serve.

Protein 24 grams | Carbs 43 grams | Calories 317

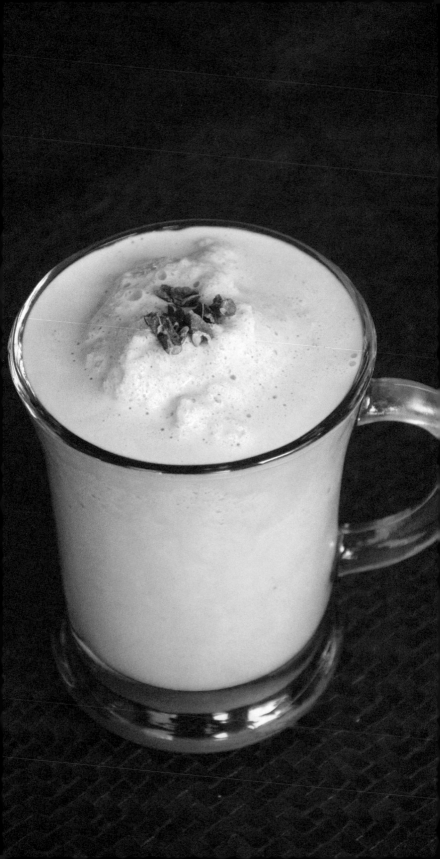

VANILLA COFFEE SHAKE

5.3 ounces vanilla Greek yogurt
1 scoop vanilla protein powder
2 teaspoons espresso powder

¼ cup 2% milk
1 cup ice

1. Add all ingredients to a blender and blend until smooth.
2. Pour into glass.
3. Serve.

Protein 43 grams | Carbs 9 grams | Calories 149

Need that jolt of coffee in the morning? This Vanilla Coffee Shake will open your eyes and get your engines revving for the day. It's loaded with protein so it will keep you going long after you've finished its icy cold goodness.

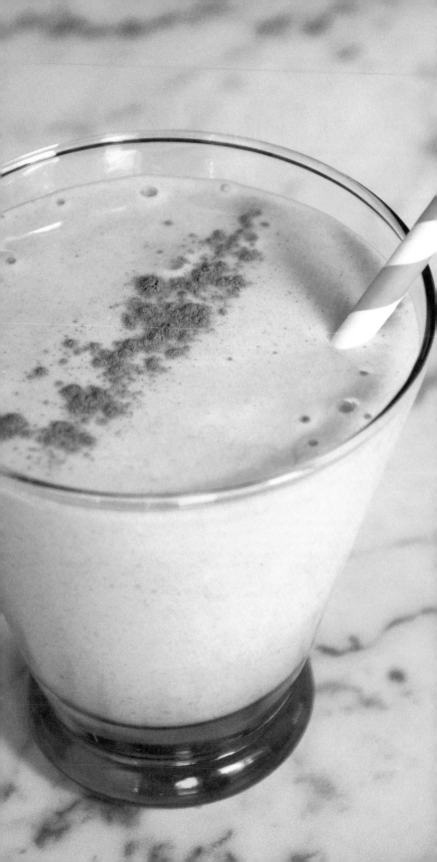

CINNAMON ROLL SHAKE

1 medium banana, cut into chunks and frozen
2 tablespoons old-fashioned rolled oats
1 scoop vanilla protein powder
1 tablespoon sugar-free vanilla pudding mix

½ teaspoon ground cinnamon
¼ teaspoon vanilla extract
¾ cup unsweetened cashew milk
Very small pinch kosher salt

1. Add all ingredients to a blender and blend until smooth.
2. Pour into glass.
3. Serve.

Protein 29 grams | Carbs 43 grams | Calories 292

Thought cinnamon rolls only came in boxes from a mall kiosk? This Cinnamon Roll Shake has the richness and flavor of your favorite cinnamon roll without all the fat and calories. You can't miss the cinnamon, since there's a good amount of it in this shake. And that vanilla glaze flavor comes through from the pudding mix.

CHOCOLATE PEANUT BUTTER SHAKE

1 medium banana, cut into
    chunks and frozen
¼ cup powdered peanut butter
½ cup silken tofu
1 tablespoon unsweetened
    cocoa powder

1 tablespoon hemp hearts
¾ cup unsweetened cashew
    milk

1. Add all ingredients to a blender and blend until smooth.
2. Pour into glass.
3. Serve.

Protein 36 grams | Carbs 55 grams | Calories 431

This thick and creamy shake is full of chocolate and peanut butter flavor. Using powdered peanut butter in this recipe keeps the peanut flavor strong but cuts down on the fat and calories of adding regular peanut butter. This protein-packed shake is perfect for an after workout snack.

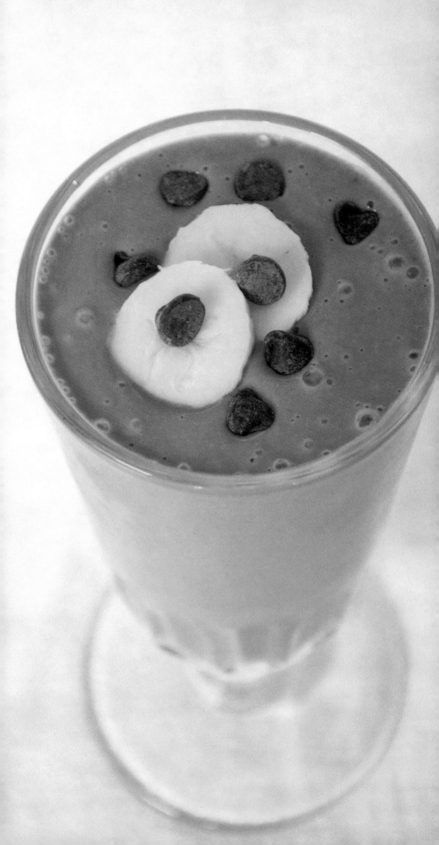

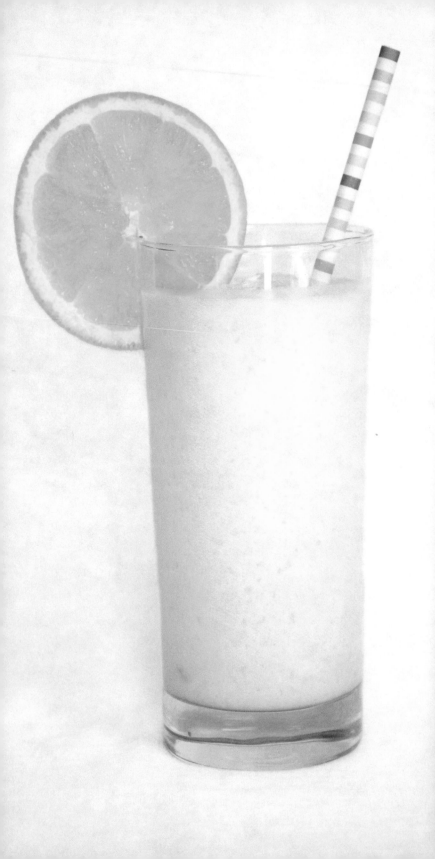

ORANGE CREAM SHAKE

½ cup low-fat 2% cottage
   cheese
½ cup silken tofu
1 navel orange, peeled and
   de-seeded

¼ teaspoon vanilla extract
1 cup ice cubes
1 tablespoon maple syrup
   (optional)

1. Add all ingredients to a blender and blend until smooth.
2. Pour into glass.
3. Serve.

Protein 23 grams | Carbs 23 grams | Calories 226

This cool and creamy shake is reminiscent
of those orange vanilla pops on a stick you
used to eat as a kid. But this Orange Cream
Shake is loaded with protein so it will keep
you going long after you've finished the
last sip.

BAHAMA MAMA SHAKE

¾ cup frozen pineapple
½ cup frozen mango
1 medium banana, cut into
    chunks and frozen

1 scoop vanilla protein powder
1 tablespoon hemp hearts
1 cup coconut water

---

1. Add all ingredients to a blender and blend until smooth.
2. Pour into glass.
3. Serve.

Protein 35 grams | Carbs 65 grams | Calories 398

If a tropical getaway is all you can think about, this Bahama Mama Shake will take you there—in spirit anyway. The mixture of pineapple, mango, and banana is a tropical treat for your taste buds. The protein powder in here is just the icing on the cake.

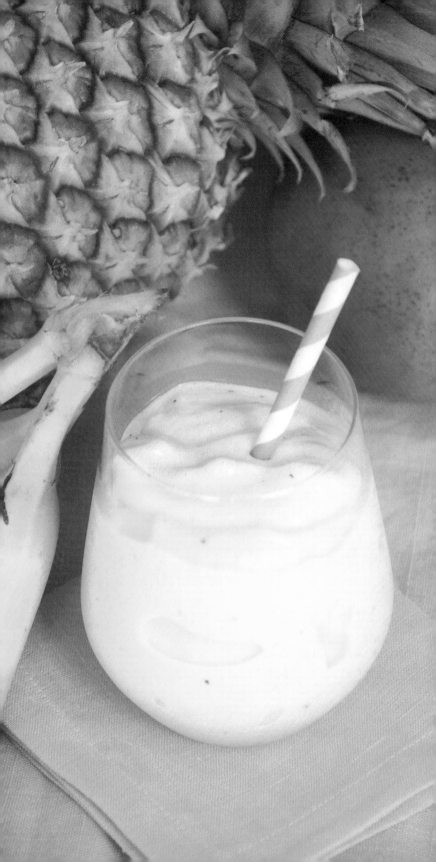

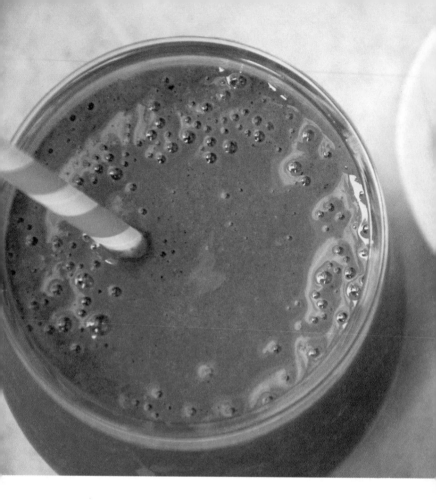

MEAN GREEN SHAKE

5.3 ounces plain Greek yogurt
1 cup frozen pineapple chunks
1 cup packed baby spinach
½ cup silken tofu

1 tablespoon organic spirulina
    powder
¾ cup unsweetened cashew
    milk

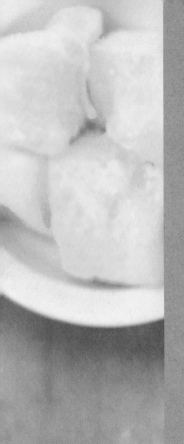

Don't be fooled by the name . . . this Mean Green Shake is actually quite nice. The pineapple gives it a pleasant sweetness and you can't even taste the spinach. So you get your protein and your greens all at the same time.

1. Add all ingredients to a blender and blend until smooth.
2. Pour into glass.
3. Serve.

Protein 31 grams | Carbs 30 grams | Calories 201

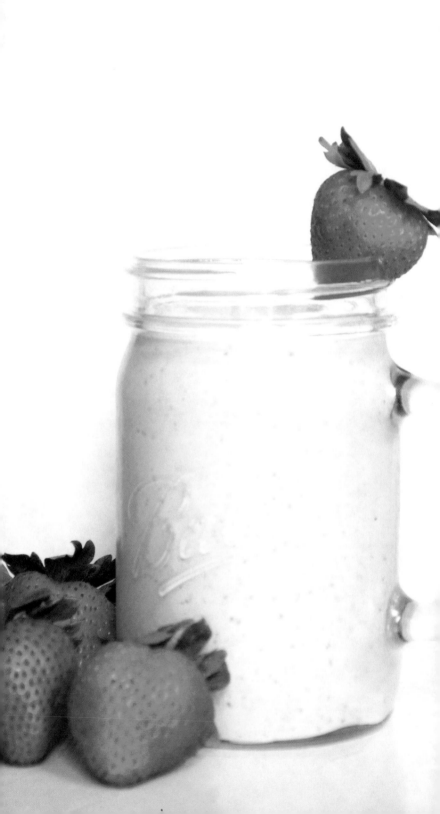

STRAWBERRY SHORTCAKE SHAKE

1 cup frozen strawberries
5.3 ounces vanilla Greek yogurt
1 scoop vanilla protein powder

¼ cup old-fashioned rolled oats
1 cup unsweetened cashew
  milk

1. Add all ingredients to a blender and blend until smooth.
2. Pour into glass.
3. Serve.

Protein 45 grams | Carbs 43 grams | Calories 261

Strawberry shortcake is a favorite summertime dessert. Why not enjoy a shake that tastes like that favorite dessert for breakfast or as a snack? This shake is rich in protein and has a great strawberry flavor. It tastes best when you use fresh frozen strawberries that are at their peak ripeness.

PEACHES & CREAM SHAKE

1 cup frozen peaches
5.3 ounces vanilla Greek yogurt
10 raw almonds

1 tablespoon hemp hearts
1 cup unsweetened cashew
  milk

1. Add all ingredients to a blender and blend until smooth.
2. Pour into glass.
3. Serve.

Protein 24 grams | Carbs 36 grams | Calories 212

A big bowl of peaches with a touch of cream poured over them is a delicious snack. This shake will give you that same great flavor but with a lot more protein to help fuel you through your day. The vanilla flavor in this shake is what I think puts it over the top.

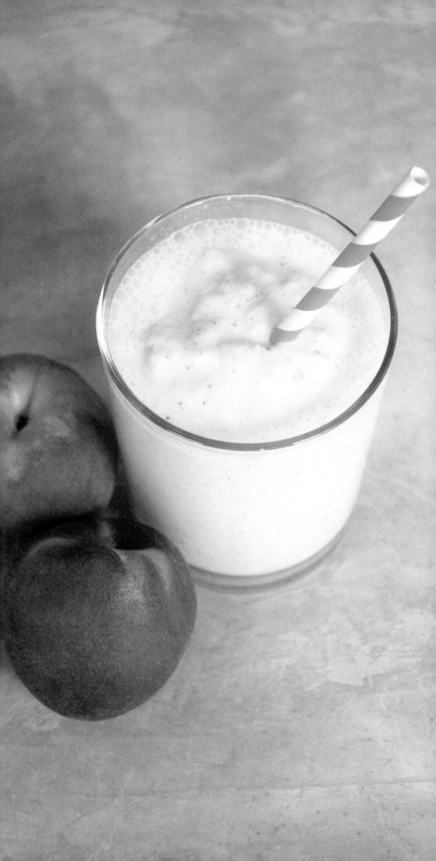

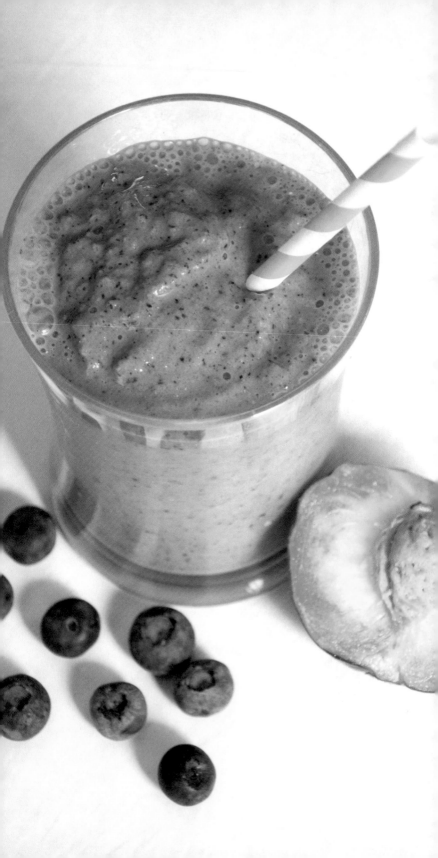

PEACHY KEEN SHAKE

1 cup frozen peaches
½ cup frozen blueberries
5.3 ounces plain Greek yogurt

1 scoop unsweetened unflavored protein powder
1 cup unsweetened cashew milk

1. Add all ingredients to a blender and blend until smooth.
2. Pour into glass.
3. Serve.

Protein 36 grams | Carbs 36 grams | Calories 221

Peaches and blueberries go together really well, so they've been paired up in this delicious high-protein shake. Thanks to the blueberries, this shake is also high in antioxidants—and the peaches make it a good source of vitamin C.

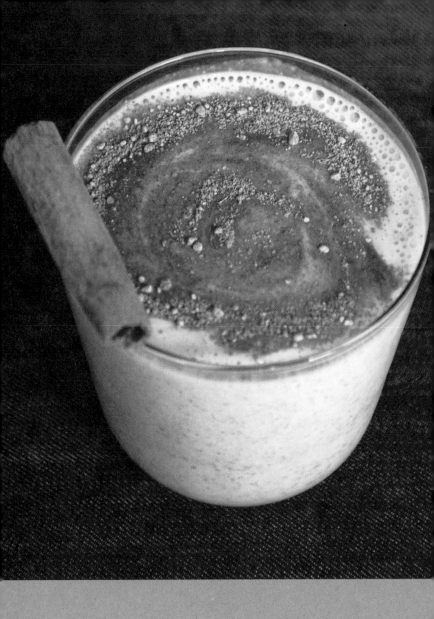

The aromatic spices that go into making your favorite chai drink work perfectly in this subtly spiced shake. Combined with the vanilla Greek yogurt, the spices take on a sweeter flavor that is a great way to start your day without having to stop at your favorite coffee shop.

CHAI SHAKE

5.3 ounces vanilla Greek yogurt
½ teaspoon ground cinnamon
¼ teaspoon ground cardamom
Small pinch ground cloves
⅛ teaspoon ground ginger
⅛ teaspoon ground allspice

1 tablespoon hemp hearts
1 tablespoon chia seeds
1 medium banana, cut into
    chunks and frozen
½ cup unsweetened cashew
    milk

1. Add all ingredients to a blender and blend until smooth.
2. Pour into glass.
3. Serve.

Protein 23 grams | Carbs 50 grams | Calories 226

PEANUT HONEY SHAKE

5.3 ounces plain Greek yogurt
2 tablespoons honey (plus more
    for drizzling in glass)
½ cup powdered peanut butter
1 tablespoon chia seeds

1 medium banana, cut into
    chunks and frozen
½ cup unsweetened cashew
    milk

---

1. Add all ingredients to a blender and blend until smooth.
2. Pour into glass.
3. Serve.

Protein 40 grams | Carbs 89 grams | Calories 490

If you love peanut butter, you're really going to like this Peanut Honey Shake. It's rich with peanut flavor and gets its sweetness from the honey. To get even more honey flavor, drizzle the inside of the glass with honey before pouring the shake into the glass. It also makes for a pretty presentation.

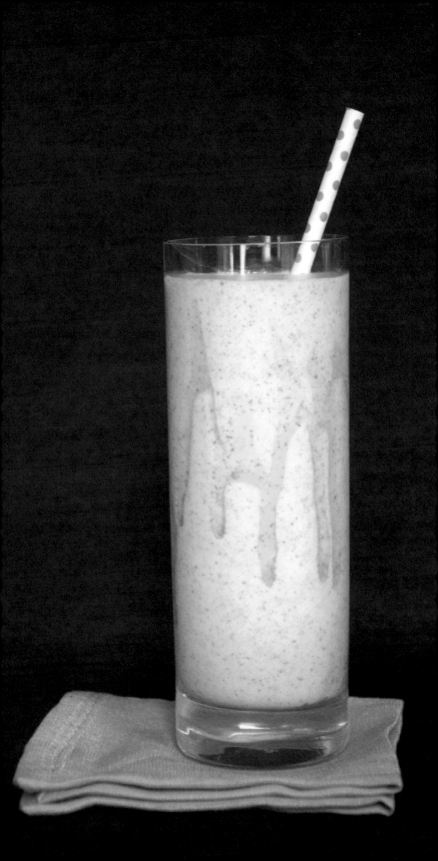

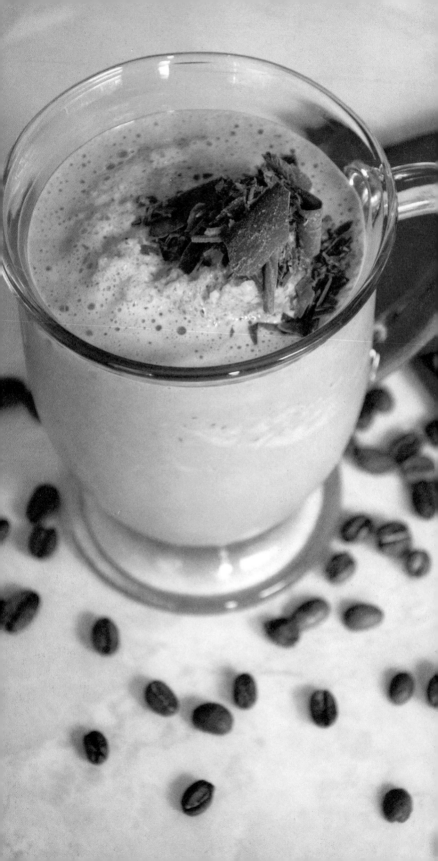

MOCHA SHAKE

5.3 ounces plain Greek yogurt
1 scoop chocolate protein
 powder
1½ teaspoons espresso powder

½ cup 2% milk
1 cup ice
1 tablespoon maple syrup
 (optional)

---

1. Add all ingredients to a blender and blend until smooth.
2. Pour into glass.
3. Serve.

Protein 36 grams | Carbs 20 grams | Calories 219

This not-too-sweet Mocha Shake will definitely get your eyes open in the morning, or keep them perky mid-afternoon. The espresso powder gives you a stronger coffee flavor than using some of your regular morning java. Because it's blended with ice, it's a perfect hot-weather drink.

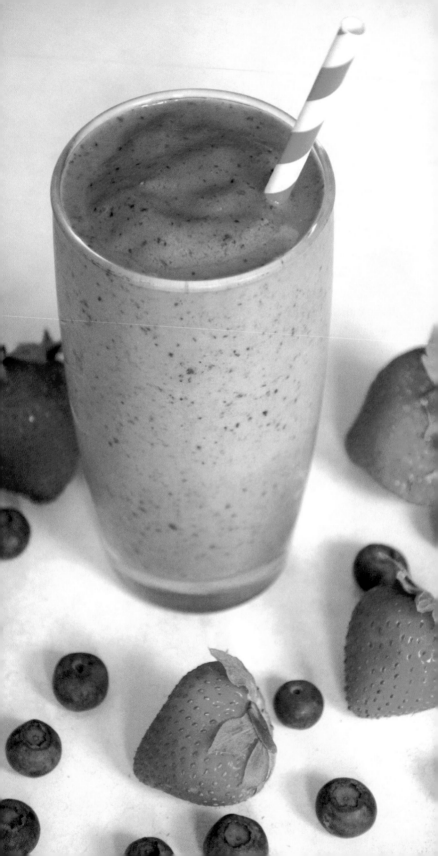

BERRY AÇAÍ SHAKE

5.3 ounces plain Greek yogurt
100-gram pack frozen açaí
  berry puree
1½ cups frozen strawberries
½ cup frozen blueberries

1 scoop unflavored, unsweetened protein powder
1¼ cups unsweetened cashew
  milk

---

1. Add all ingredients to a blender and blend until smooth.
2. Pour into glass.
3. Serve.

Protein 37 grams | Carbs 41 grams | Calories 302

This lightly sweetened shake is full of delicious fruity goodness. It's got a bit of tartness from the yogurt, which adds to the overall flavor. Talk about a shake that's full of good-for-you stuff. This shake's not only loaded with protein, but it's got antioxidants, vitamins, and fiber.

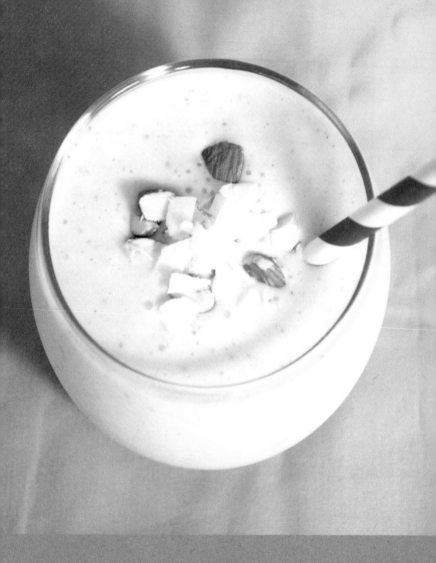

It's time to go nuts! Coconut and almond combine in this smooth and creamy shake. Coconut milk makes this rich and velvety and the almond flavor pairs really well with the sweet coconut.

ALMOND COCONUT SHAKE

ALMOND COCONUT SHAKE

5.3 ounces plain Greek yogurt
1 medium banana, cut into
  chunks and frozen
½ cup silken tofu
10 raw almonds
¼ teaspoon almond extract

2 tablespoons unsweetened
  coconut flakes
¼ cup canned coconut milk
¼ cup unsweetened cashew
  milk

1. Add all ingredients to a blender and blend until smooth.
2. Pour into glass.
3. Serve.

Protein 30 grams | Carbs 42 grams | Calories 469

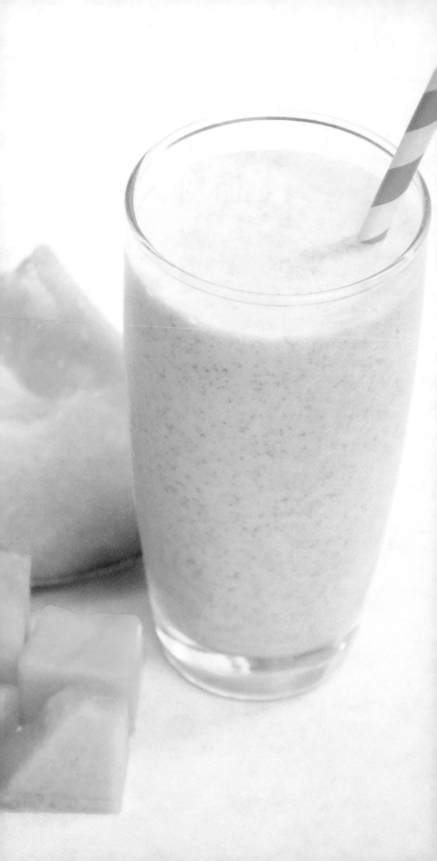

SUMMER CANTALOUPE SHAKE

5.3 ounces vanilla Greek yogurt
1 ¼ cups cantaloupe, cut into
chunks and frozen
1 tablespoon hemp hearts

1 tablespoon chia seeds
½ cup unsweetened cashew
milk

1. Add all ingredients to a blender and blend until smooth.
2. Pour into glass.
3. Serve.

Protein 23 grams | Carbs 39 grams | Calories 181

Frozen chunks of fresh cantaloupe combine with vanilla Greek yogurt in this cool and creamy shake. You get an extra shot of protein from the hemp hearts and chia seeds. You'll need to cut up your own cantaloupe for this recipe since it's almost impossible to find frozen cantaloupe. But you'll be rewarded with a great-tasting shake.

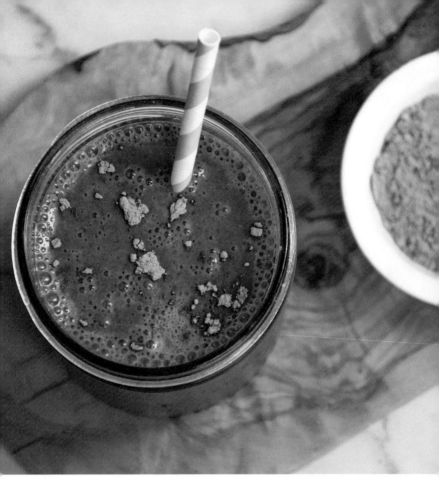

MATCHA SHAKE

5.3 ounces vanilla Greek yogurt
1 tablespoon unsweetened
   matcha powder
1 tablespoon organic spirulina
   powder

1 tablespoon hemp hearts
1 medium banana, cut into
   chunks and frozen
¾ cup unsweetened cashew
   milk

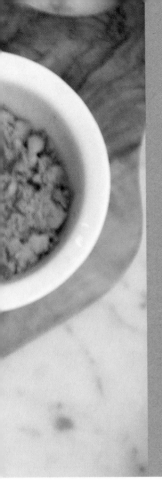

Green tea powder (matcha) pairs with vanilla in this creamy, rich shake. The vanilla mellows out the flavor of the matcha so that it's not overpowering. Adding spirulina gives you more protein and nutrients as well as that bright green color.

1. Add all ingredients to a blender and blend until smooth.
2. Pour into glass.
3. Serve.

Protein 25 grams | Carbs 54 grams | Calories 245

MATCHA SHAKE

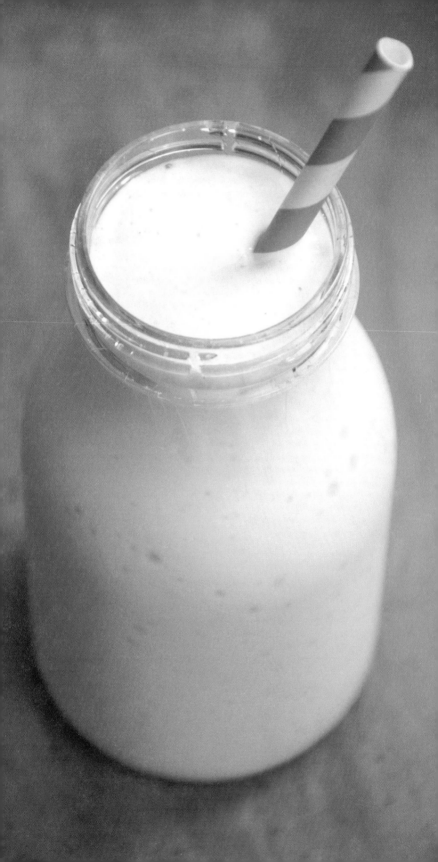

VANILLA SHAKE

5.3 ounces vanilla Greek yogurt
1 scoop vanilla protein powder
1 medium banana, cut into
    chunks and frozen

½ teaspoon vanilla extract
½ cup unsweetened cashew
    milk

1. Add all ingredients to a blender and blend until smooth.
2. Pour into glass.
3. Serve.

Protein 41 grams | Carbs 42 grams | Calories 238

If you're a vanilla fan then this shake is for you—you've got vanilla three ways in here. While you get a big punch of vanilla-flavored protein from the protein powder, you get extra from the vanilla Greek yogurt, and even more vanilla flavor from the extract.

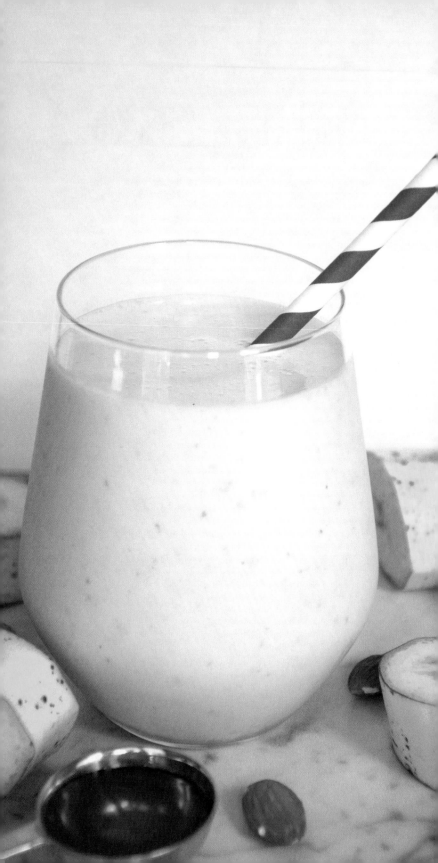

HONEY BANANA SHAKE

5.3 ounces plain Greek yogurt
¼ cup cannellini beans, drained
   and rinsed
1 medium banana, cut into
   chunks and frozen

10 raw almonds
2 tablespoons honey
½ cup unsweetened cashew
   milk

1. Add all ingredients to a blender and blend until smooth.
2. Pour into glass.
3. Serve.

Protein 22 grams | Carbs 69 grams | Calories 339

This protein-rich Honey Banana Shake is a great on-the-go breakfast that will stay with you for hours. Banana helps to protect your heart and aids in calcium absorption, which you get a good dose of from the yogurt in this shake.

BANANA OAT SHAKE

1 medium banana, cut into
  chunks and frozen
2 tablespoons old-fashioned
  rolled oats
1 tablespoon creamy peanut
  butter

1 tablespoon chia seeds
1 teaspoon honey
1 scoop unflavored, unsweetened protein powder
¾ cup unsweetened cashew
  milk

---

1. Add all ingredients to a blender and blend until smooth.
2. Pour into glass.
3. Serve.

Protein 27 grams | Carbs 53 grams | Calories 411

Bananas, peanut butter, and oatmeal come together for a delicious breakfast or a quick on-the-go snack. The protein powder adds a big dose of protein, so this shake will stay with you for a long time and not cause you to crash.

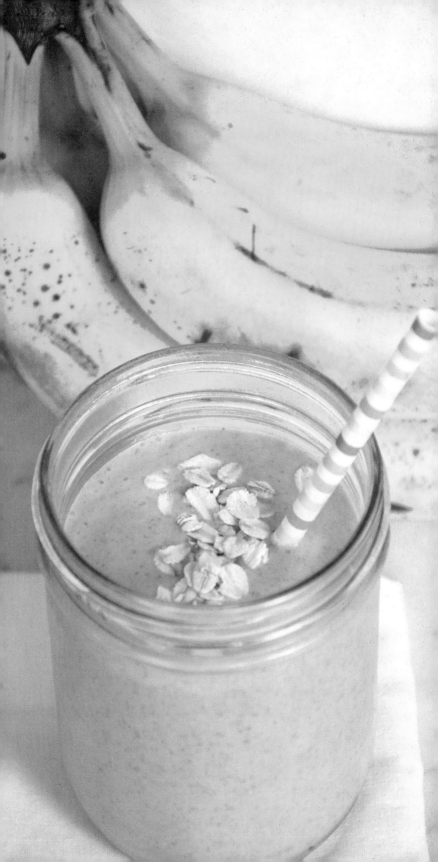

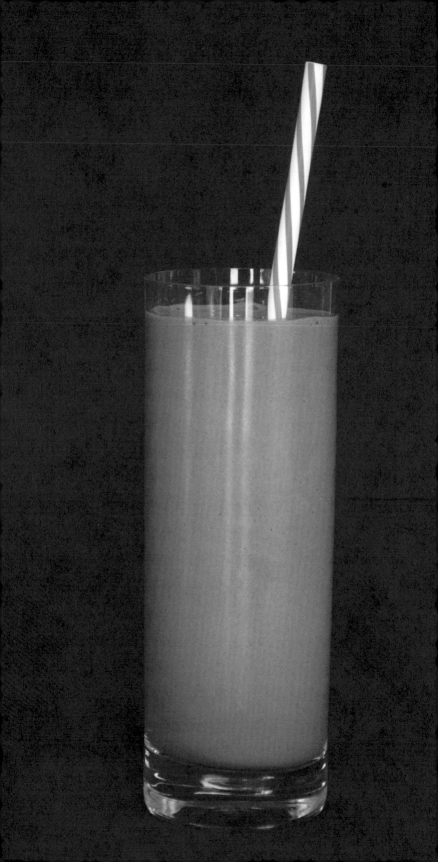

DARK CHOCOLATE PEPPERMINT SHAKE

1 medium banana, cut into
chunks and frozen
1 scoop chocolate protein
powder
1 tablespoon unsweetened
cocoa powder

½ teaspoon vanilla extract
⅛ teaspoon peppermint extract
¾ cup unsweetened cashew
milk

1. Add all ingredients to a blender and blend until smooth.
2. Pour into glass.
3. Serve.

Protein 19 grams | Carbs 40 grams | Calories 286

Can't get enough of chocolate and mint flavor combinations? This thick and rich shake is for you. You get the best of both flavor worlds here. Then there's the added bonus that it's chock full of good-for-you protein. You can choose the amount of mint you want in this shake by changing how much extract you add to the recipe.

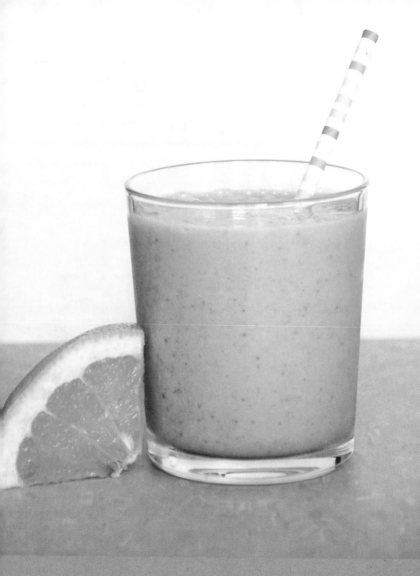

Long after those hot months have gone away and you're still looking for something to spark your taste buds like those summer drinks did, this shake comes along to save the day. The bright-tasting grapefruit pairs with the sweet taste of pineapple to make for a delicious shake. And no, you won't even taste the spinach.

GRAPEFRUIT SQUEEZE SHAKE

GRAPEFRUIT SQUEEZE SHAKE

1 pink grapefruit, peeled and seeded
1 cup frozen pineapple
1 medium banana, cut into chunks and frozen
¼ cup cannellini beans, drained and rinsed

1 scoop unflavored, unsweetened protein powder
1 cup packed baby spinach
¾ cup unsweetened cashew milk

1. Add all ingredients to a blender and blend until smooth.
2. Pour into glass.
3. Serve.

Protein 23 grams | Carbs 54 grams | Calories 298

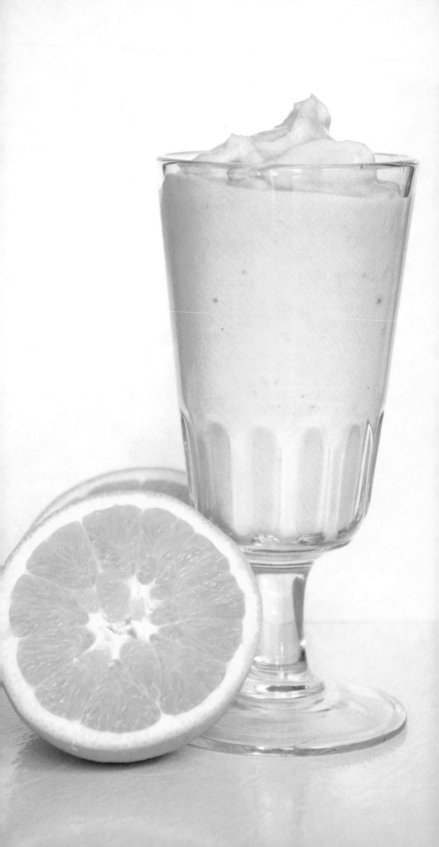

ORANGE MANGO SHAKE

5.3 ounces plain Greek yogurt
1 medium banana, cut into
   chunks and frozen
1 cup frozen mango pieces
1 navel orange, peeled and
   de-seeded

1 scoop unflavored, unsweetened protein powder
¾ cup unsweetened cashew
   milk

1. Add all ingredients to a blender and blend until smooth.
2. Pour into glass.
3. Serve.

Protein 38 grams | Carbs 76 grams | Calories 371

A similar shake is on a famous chain's menu and this one tastes a whole lot like it. But this one won't cost you as much money if you make it yourself. The shake is also loaded with way more protein than that other one. So break out the blender and make yourself this delicious shake and laugh at everyone else spending their money.

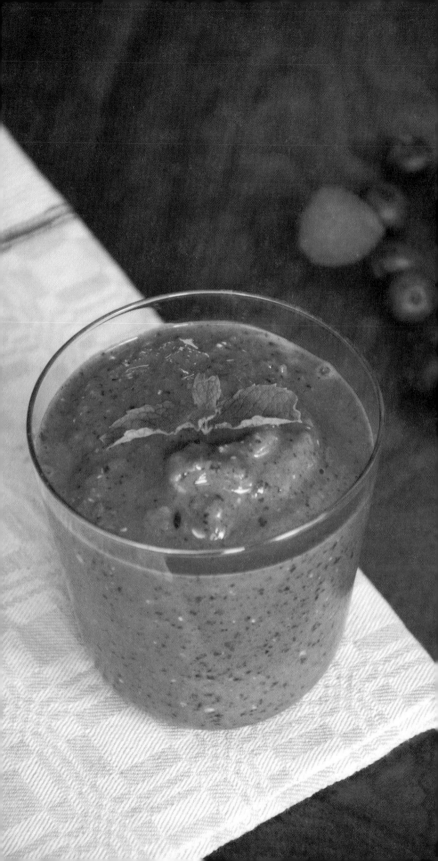

BERRY OAT SHAKE

5.3 ounces plain Greek yogurt
½ cup frozen blueberries
¼ cup frozen raspberries
5 frozen strawberries
¼ cup cannellini beans, drained
  and rinsed

2 tablespoons old-fashioned
  rolled oats
1 teaspoon honey
1 cup unsweetened cashew
  milk

1. Add all ingredients to a blender and blend until smooth.
2. Pour into glass.
3. Serve.

Protein 22 grams | Carbs 43 grams | Calories 188

Oatmeal is a very popular item for breakfast and many times we top it with berries. This time it's the berries' turn to be the main dish and the oatmeal just goes along for the ride. This shake gets its sweetness from the berries but gets a little help from some honey. You can leave that out if you don't want it quite as sweet.

PB&J SHAKE

1 medium banana, cut into chunks and frozen
½ cup frozen strawberries
1 tablespoon creamy peanut butter

1 scoop vanilla protein powder
1 tablespoon flax seeds
¾ cup unsweetened cashew milk

1. Add all ingredients to a blender and blend until smooth.
2. Pour into glass.
3. Serve.

Protein 33 grams | Carbs 40 grams | Calories 406

Get your morning started off right by bringing out your inner kid with this PB&J Shake. You may be missing the bread, but you won't be missing the peanut butter and fruit flavor. Plus this shake has lots of protein to fill you up.

Start your day off with a big dose of protein and a breakfast you can take on the go.

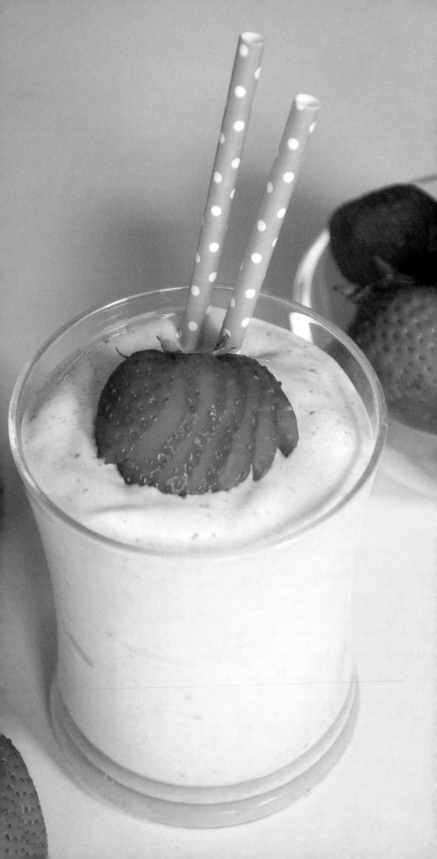

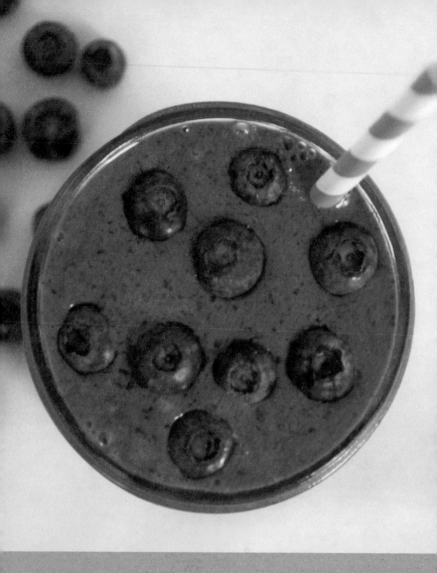

This Purple Power Shake is filling from the protein and fiber in it. Its deep purple color is just an added bonus as are the calcium and antioxidants found in this great shake.

PURPLE POWER SHAKE

PURPLE POWER
SHAKE

5.3 ounces vanilla Greek yogurt
1 tablespoon maca powder
1 cup frozen blueberries
100-gram pack frozen açaí
    berry puree

1 scoop unflavored, unsweet-
    ened protein powder
1 teaspoon maple syrup
½ cup ice
¾ cup coconut water

1. Add all ingredients to a blender and blend until smooth.
2. Pour into glass.
3. Serve.

Protein 35 grams | Carbs 56 grams | Calories 314

LEMON MERINGUE SHAKE

¼ cup raw cashews, soaked in water overnight

½ cup low-fat 2% cottage cheese

1 scoop vanilla protein powder

½ teaspoon honey

1 medium banana, cut into chunks and frozen

Juice of ½ lemon

½ teaspoon lemon zest

½ cup unsweetened cashew milk

1. Drain cashews.
2. Add all ingredients to a blender and blend until smooth.
3. Pour into glass.
4. Serve.

Protein 46 grams | Carbs 45 grams | Calories 516

Don't you just love a big slice of lemon meringue pie when it's hot outside? This shake lets you enjoy all those great lemony flavors while choosing a healthier option. This shake is creamy and lemony with just the right amount of pucker and sweet.

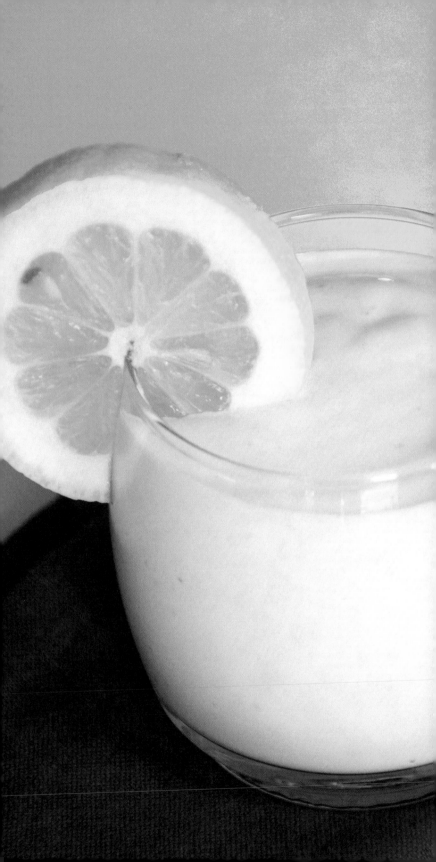

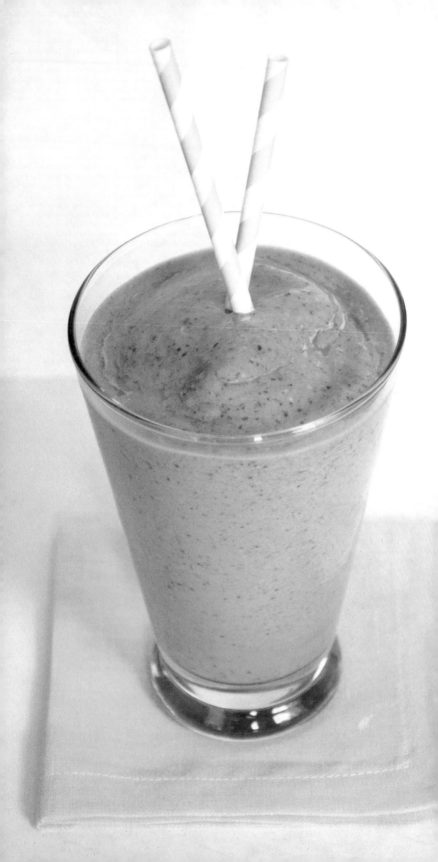

GREEN WARRIOR SHAKE

½ cup frozen pineapple chunks
1 medium banana, cut into
  chunks and frozen
10 raw almonds
1 cup packed baby spinach
½ small avocado, peeled and
  pitted

1 scoop vanilla protein powder
½ teaspoon organic spirulina
  powder
1 cup unsweetened cashew
  milk

1. Add all ingredients to a blender and blend until smooth.
2. Pour into glass.
3. Serve.

Protein 36 grams | Carbs 50 grams | Calories 491

There's something about a green shake that lets you know you must be getting something that's good for you. This shake isn't just about the green though—it tastes really good too. It has spinach and spirulina for all those healthy nutrients, pineapple and banana for sweetness, and avocado for some healthy fats. Oh, and don't forget the punch of protein.

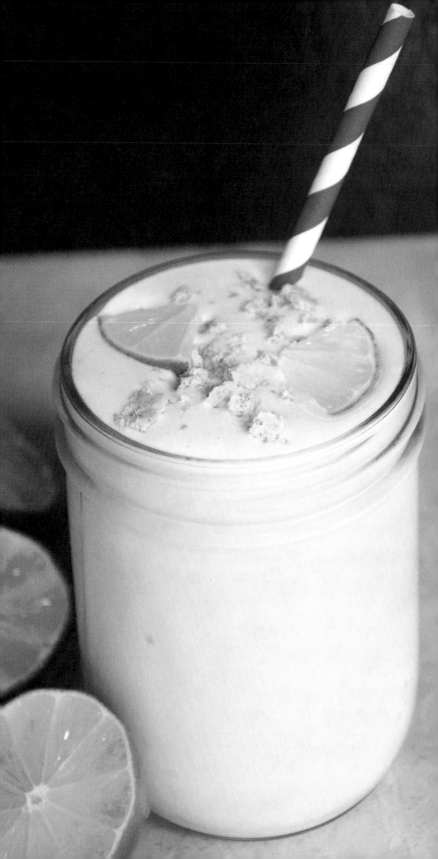

KEY LIME PIE SHAKE

5.3 ounces plain Greek yogurt
1 scoop vanilla protein powder
1 teaspoon unsweetened lime
  Jell-O mix
1 medium banana, cut into
  chunks and frozen

½ teaspoon maple syrup
½ cup unsweetened cashew
  milk

1. Add all ingredients to a blender and blend until smooth.
2. Pour into glass.
3. Serve.

Protein 42 grams | Carbs 40 grams | Calories 249

This Key Lime Pie Shake has all the best parts of key lime pie but better. It's tangy and sweet and a great source of protein. Why not start your day off with dessert? You can when it's this good for you.

* Note: **Boldface** indicates illustrations